THE

BETTER

BACK

BOOK

MICHAEL D. WOLF, Ph.D. & JULIE DAVIS

Contemporary Books, Inc.
Chicago

Library of Congress Cataloging in Publication Data

Wolf, Michael D.
   The better back book.

   Includes index.
   1. Back—Care and hygiene.   2. Exercise therapy.
3. Backache—Prevention.   I. Davis, Julie, 1956–
II. Title.
RD768.W65   1984   617'.56052   83-27308
ISBN 0-8092-5443-3

All photos © Marti Cohen-Wolf

Published by Contemporary Books, Inc.
180 North Michigan Avenue, Chicago, Illinois 60601
Manufactured in the United States of America
Library of Congress Catalog Number: 83-27308
International Standard Book Number: 0-8092-5443-3

Published simultaneously in Canada by Beaverbooks, Ltd.
195 Allstate Parkway, Valleywood Business Park
Markham, Ontario L3R 4T8 Canada

CONTENTS

FOREWORD

Low back pain shows no favorites, striking Olympic athletes just as it can executives and homemakers. In an active and stress-filled American society, the need for an intelligent prevention and care program could not be more critical.

The Better Back Book provides just such a program, emphasizing prevention through intelligent stretching, exercise, and movement. Sections on medical practitioners and therapeutic approaches to back rehabilitation provide the reader with an unbiased guide to back care.

I recommend this book highly, no matter what type of athlete you might be—Olympic, weekend, or armchair.

Irving Dardik, M.D.
Chairman, U.S. Olympic Committee, Sports Medicine Council

ACKNOWLEDGMENTS

Special thanks to the following friends who helped make this book possible:

Marti Cohen-Wolf, our photographer (and my wife), who shot two books and produced two multi-image slide shows in one very crazy six-week period.

Our tireless and ever-smiling model Brenda Bernhardt Frasca, now a veteran of three Contemporary Books projects.

Our ace stylist/makeup/hair designer Daphne White.

Harold Hein of International Furniture Industries, Inc., New York City, who supplied the Giroflex chair seen in Chapter Four.

The four gracious and capable physicians we interviewed to produce Chapter 3:

Vincent K. McInerney, M.D., Director of Orthopedic Education and Sportsmedicine/Human Performance Center at St. Joseph's Hospital and Medical Center, Paterson, New Jersey.

Joan J. McInerney, M.D., Orthopedic Surgeon, Lakeland, Florida.

Michael M. Silverman, D.O., Assistant Clinical Professor of Osteopathic Medicine at the New Jersey College of Medicine and Dentistry, and a licensed/board certified Osteopathic Physician in private practice in River Vale, New Jersey.

Charles S. Berg, D.C., Teaching Faculty of the New York Chiropractic College, and a licensed Chiropractic Physician in private practice in River Vale, New Jersey.

We could not have found four better representatives of their health care specialties.

1

INTRODUCTION: PREVENTION, NOT CURE

Protecting the physical integrity of the back is a vital yet often neglected part of achieving good health. Consider that, at one time or another, everyone will experience some form of back discomfort. You might feel that certain twinge that comes from bending the wrong way to pick up a book or tie a shoe; you might wake up with that nagging ache that takes a few minutes, every morning, to work itself out; or perhaps you will suffer an assault to the back that requires professional attention. There's no doubt that working to avoid a problem back makes sense.

Creating a healthy back through good comportment and the right fitness program is a must for everyone, regardless of age, whether you think of yourself as active or sedentary. The irony of most fitness plans is that in your quest to become physically fit, you can do yourself more harm than good if you are an uninformed athlete. Indeed, some of the most common exercises can harm the back. Our program will offer you the good health you want as well as protect you from sports injuries: a better back (and body) through prevention.

For those who have a bad back, we'll guide you to the right practitioner and, after medical treatment, will teach you to exercise your back in a way that will prevent a relapse. What we will not tell you to do is attempt to diagnose your own condition; that is the most dangerous mistake you could make. Skipping necessary medical treatment or prescribing it yourself will take you from bad to worse. Only the proper therapy coupled with the proper exercise and stretching routine will give you the terrific all-over feeling you want.

HOW TO USE THIS BOOK

To give yourself a strong foundation of knowledge from which to judge your general health, read the following chapter on back pain. If you feel that you are bothered by backache, read Chapter 3 to learn about the various practitioners and options available to you. Also read Chapter 4 to learn how to hold and move your body to limit the damage done to your back. After treatment, you may begin the stretching and exercise program.

If you are in good shape and are interested in preventing any problems as you exercise, start the program outlined in chapters 5 and 6, but only after mastering the basics of comportment in Chapter 4.

If you have already had medical treatment and have resisted renewing an exercise program, start practicing the stretches in Chapter 5 as well as the guidelines in Chapter 4. These movements will give you the flexibility and assurance to renew a more active exercise plan, usually within three weeks.

Above all, tailor the information to your best use and start on a positive course of action right away.

2

WHAT IS BACK PAIN?

ANATOMY "101"

To understand back pain, it is important to first have a general understanding of your body. Your body is supported by the spine, a complex network of bones—notably the *vertebrae* and *interlocking joints*—and tissue. Think of the spine as a great three-dimensional "S," an important image. Maintaining the curves of that "S" and the lower curve—known as the *lumbar* spine—will mean the difference between a healthy back and one that is more susceptible to injury and internal damage.

Though the vertebrae and the interlocking joints make up the structure of the spine, the other components are equally crucial to good health. The *discs,* made up of cartilage surrounding soft matter, lie between each vertebra and act as shock absorbers to the spine as you bend, twist, or turn. The *spinal cord* itself, a soft, jelly-like mass, runs through the interlocking joints, enclosing the nerves that relay orders from the brain to the other parts of the body.

Working with these four major components are *muscles* and *ligaments* that support the spine. Interestingly, not only back

3

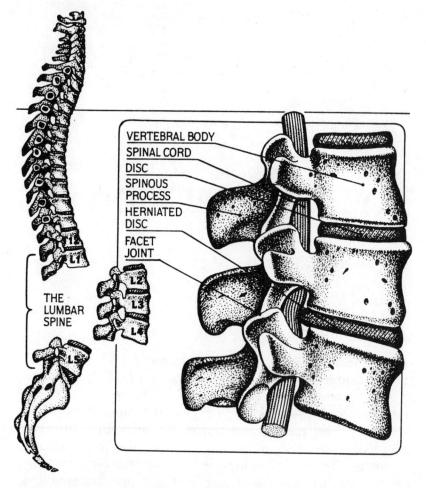

VERTEBRAL BODY
SPINAL CORD
DISC
SPINOUS PROCESS
HERNIATED DISC
FACET JOINT

THE LUMBAR SPINE

L1
L2
L3
L4
L5

An overall view of the spine and a detailed view of the all-important lumbar region featuring healthy discs as well as a herniated one. Illustration reprinted courtesy of Glenbrook Laboratories, a division of the Bayer Company.

muscles affect the back; the abdominals do as well. And the physical integrity (or good condition) of other parts of the body, such as the weight-bearing joints of the ankles, knees, and hips, helps take the load off the back.

As you can see, the spine is to be protected at all costs, for equal to its importance in the body is the chance that it may be damaged.

WHAT IS BACK PAIN?

There can be no doubt that in such an anatomically complex structure, a wide variety of problems—with an equally wide variety of causes—can occur. The vast majority of back problems are explained by: (1) strains and sprains of the muscles and ligaments, and (2) herniated discs—commonly, though incorrectly described as *slipped* discs. (Of course, back pain can be a signal of other, more serious ailments; for this reason, medical attention should never be put off.)

When the trouble centers on muscles and ligaments, the pain is most likely localized in the lower back region. Causes can include:

- poor posture
- lack of exercise
- obesity (particularly a heavy "gut" that pulls the spine forward)
- muscles contracted for a prolonged period of time
- emotional tension and mental stress
- a trauma or physical assault stemming from an injury or accident
- moving too quickly or suddenly into an unusual position such as bending the wrong way
- holding an unusual position for too long, and getting out of it too quickly as well
- stress and build-up of muscular tension from lifting a heavy object incorrectly and repeatedly over the long term.

Note that the severity of the pain will vary, depending on the actual insult to the body.

Each or any combination of these causes can, over a long period of time, add up to a major trauma and cause the herniated disc condition. When the spine is continually misused, the resulting misalignment of vertebrae causes a rupturing of a disc; the disc presses backward on the spinal cord or diagonally outward on the nerves, creating pain that spreads to other parts of the body. The most prevalent condition is called sciatica: the disc presses on the sciatic nerve that runs through both legs, the route this pain travels.

The chief way to distinguish muscular from disc pain is to

remember that *muscular pain is localized* and often responds to the home therapies described in the next section. *Disc conditions engender pain that radiates* down the legs, signaling serious nerve involvement. Tingling and numbness are other symptoms that demand immediate medical attention because (1) a ruptured disc cannot readily heal itself, and (2) the situation will worsen with every successive incorrect movement you make. Therefore, if you experience a pain so severe that you are worried, or one which home therapies do not help within a 24- to 48-hour period, the condition should be considered serious enough to warrant a practitioner's attention.

A few words to the wise: never try to self-diagnose or self-treat a back problem. The science of back medicine can be, at worst, inaccurate even in the hands of the most skilled practitioner. Not enough research has been done on the various therapies, drugs, and other treatments available (which is why there are so many to choose from: no one yet knows which is best). If a medical practitioner is not infallible when it comes to diagnosing your ailment, you certainly have far less chance of calling it correctly. Use common sense and seek a variety of professional advice from various segments of the medical community to help you make the right choice.

The following therapies include home treatments that have been helpful in many minor cases of muscular pain, as well as office treatments and other options for this and disc ailments.

PHYSICAL THERAPIES: TREATMENTS FOR RELIEVING/ CORRECTING BACK PAIN

HOME THERAPIES: TO BE USED FOR MUSCULAR ACHE ONLY

The three-step procedure that offers the most relief is called AIM—aspirin, ice, and massage. Let's explore them step by step.

Aspirin

Take aspirin immediately for its anti-inflammatory action—

aching muscles are inflamed muscles. If aspirin doesn't agree with you, try a nonaspirin pain reliever. Aspirin or analgesic cream (another type of anti-inflammatory agent) should be used in conjunction with massage. An ointment such as Aspercreme is also helpful if the heat effect reaches deep enough under the skin to warm tissues.

Ice

Ice breaks the pain cycle of a spasm. When a muscle is subjected to assault, a reflex contraction occurs to stop you from straining the muscle further. As this contraction gets tighter, you experience more pain; with added pain, more contractions occur in surrounding muscles. The four-stage action of ice stops this cycle. The easiest way to apply ice is with a homemade ice pack. Place a Styrofoam cup filled with water in the freezer (it makes sense to always have one on hand). To use it, simply peel away an inch or so of the Styrofoam to expose the round surface of ice. Now you're ready to apply it (or have it applied for you, if you are the one in pain).

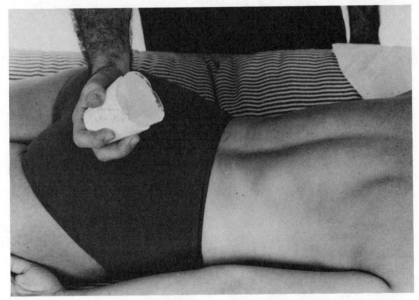

Peel away the Styrofoam as needed to expose the surface of the ice.

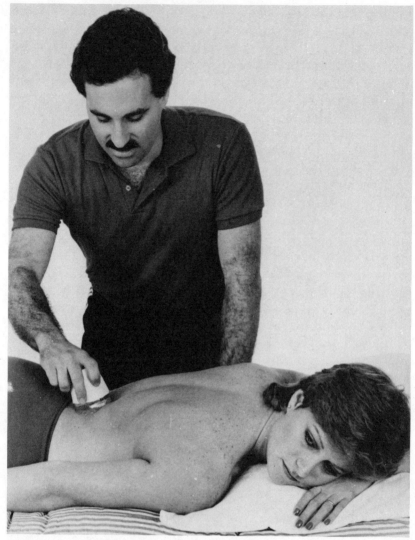

Always apply the ice cup in a circular motion.

Always apply the ice in small circles over the affected area of the back—never hold the ice in one place. When you first apply the ice, there is a cold sensation; this is the first stage. After a few minutes, an ache will be felt; this is the second stage. After five minutes, there will be a burning sensation;

stage three. Remove the ice for one to two minutes. Then return the ice to the affected area and continue the circular motion until numbness, the fourth and most crucial stage, is felt. The entire procedure should last no more than eight minutes for a small area and ten minutes for a larger area. This is how long it takes the cold to reach deep into the muscles.

An alternative to the ice cup is a plastic bag filled with ice cubes. Wrap it all in a thin, wet cloth and place it over the affected area. Because the ice is not directly on the skin, the bag and towel may be left in place until the numbness stage is reached, in about 20 to 30 minutes.

Massage

A light, hands-on massage may be used as a follow-up after the ice treatment. This helps to relieve tension—mental as well as muscular. It should be gentle, not a full Swedish massage, which calls for too much manipulation for a sore back.

If the pain has subsided, light stretching, using a small range of motion as described in Chapter 5 can be attempted. However, stretching and exercise per se are not to be used as first aids.

Heat Therapy

Although the ice treatment should be your first choice, especially in the case of a muscle spasm, individual response is unpredictable—one of your muscles might very well respond to the cold, while another won't. If, after a few minutes, you find that you are getting no relief from the ice, and more importantly, the ice is worsening your pain, stop. Try heat, using an analgesic ointment via massage and/or a heating pad. Some have found that alternating the ice cube bag and the heating pad every few minutes also provides relief.

Muscular aches will respond in anywhere from twenty minutes to several days of treatment. Again, if your pain is severe, or if it is a nagging pain that doesn't lessen after 48 hours, consult a professional immediately.

A Word About Gravity Boots

One home therapy you should avoid is the use of gravity boots. Ever since Richard Gere's famous sit-ups in the film *American Gigolo,* gravity boots, or *inversion systems,* have captured the imagination of the fitness seeker. The idea behind inversion is to decompress a compressed spinal column by hanging upside down. The system is based on the theory of traction that has helped many. However, the problem is not with gravity boots per se, but with eager users who prescribe the treatment for themselves (usually after a session of self-diagnosis). As a result, gravity boots have had a serious effect on the public—so much so that for every patient who has been successfully helped by an inversion system there is someone who became a patient as a result of their unsupervised use. Gravity boots have their place among back therapies, but please let your specialist be the judge of their potential usefulness in your individual treatment.

MEDICAL MODALITIES: THERAPIES FROM A PRACTITIONER

Various back specialists have a wide variety of modalities, or therapies, to choose from. A lot depends on the type of doctor who is treating you (see Chapter 3 for a more detailed discussion of the philosophy behind the chiropractor's, the osteopath's, and the orthopedist's treatment), as well as the type of ailment.

Ultrasound uses sound waves to drive a balm or analgesic cream deeper into the tissues via a plastic wand with rounded head to relax a muscle spasm.

Electrical stimulation is another form of therapy to relax muscles and increase healing blood flow.

Drug therapy can help muscular problems but cannot correct trouble with discs. Though doctors prescribe pills, it is often the pharmacist who is most familiar with their indications and side effects. Never take a drug without fully understanding it—your pharmacist should be consulted to supplement your practitioner's guidelines.

Physical manipulation by an osteopath, a chiropractor, or a physical therapist is a noninvasive (nonsurgical) technique used to realign the vertebrae and discs. This is a generally safe procedure and should always be investigated before considering surgery.

Traction is a mechanical form of realignment performed under clinical, supervised conditions. Again, do not attempt your own brand of gravity-boot traction without medical guidance.

Enzyme injections. The injection of enzymes that will shrink the disc is often the last choice before surgery. The most popular enzyme, chymopapain, has a 70%+ success rate, but can cause numerous side effects.

Surgery should be your last option, only after you have exhausted all other forms of treatment. It is a serious operation and does not carry any guarantees; you should consider it only after manipulation has been discounted.

RESUMING EXERCISE AFTER TREATMENT

For all but the slightest muscle spasms that you can treat at home, you'll need a medical OK to resume (or to finally begin) an exercise program. But chances are that the very M.D. who suggests you exercise and even tells you when to begin *won't* know what the right program for a better back is. The reason for this is simple: with the thousands of hours of life-saving procedures that must be learned, there is no time (or little enough) for disease-prevention training. (Practitioners like the osteopath and the chiropractor may have a better idea of what to tell you because of the slightly different emphasis of their training.)

We recommend beginning with our stretching plan in Chapter 4—the easiest stretches at first, with the shortest holding time and the least amount of reps. Your body will tell you when you're ready to add on. If you feel any pain or even discomfort, stop: you need more time to heal.

3

CHOOSING A PRACTITIONER

Treatment for disorders of the back, stemming from muscle/ ligament damage to trauma to diseases of the spinal column and discs, are quite varied. Certain therapies are available from each of the three important practitioners discussed in this chapter. Each practitioner's training and philosophy is unique and their potential benefits to the patient will depend on the condition requiring medical attention.

When trying to choose between these practitioners, bear in mind that most medical doctors are still being trained to treat sickness, not to maintain health. If we could measure good health on a scale, with 10 being perfect health, 0 being average health, and –10 being sickness, you might say that most physicians are taught to take you to 0, but they don't know how to take you beyond that to 10 (primarily because many medical schools haven't fit that into their curricula yet). There are times when a surgeon is needed, when his expertise is vital. But he is no longer the only healer who can correct a painful problem.

As you read the following profiles, treat yourself to an open mind when considering practitioners whose work may as yet be unfamiliar to you. At the right time, for the right patient (with the wrong back) any one of them might be right.

THE CHIROPRACTOR

Chiropractic is the field of healing that studies the body's system of nerves and its relationship to the mechanical functions of the spine from a structural point of view. The chiropractor is a trained practitioner and a licensed physician. He is skilled in hands-on spinal manipulation as the primary means of not only treating, but of ultimately correcting a low back problem. He believes that disease may be caused or aggravated by disturbances in the nervous system and that these disturbances have a probable root in misalignments of the musculo-skeletal structure of the body. When structure is affected, function is affected.

The chiropractor's primary goal, once pain is relieved, is to correct the anatomical condition responsible for the trouble, and not just treat its symptoms. If not, the problem will simply keep reoccurring.

The chiropractor sees specific assaults as being the cause of a low back condition. Low back pain is often due to accidents, such as falling off a bike, or to trauma, one as unsuspected as that created by sliding down a flight of stairs on one's bottom as a child. These "insults" create, over time, biomechanical problems such as misalignments, that might not surface until much later. The chiropractor tries to undo the effects of years of wear and tear through treatment.

The chiropractor is a great believer in prevention and early detection, and often advises putting children through an examination early in life before the body sends out its last defense signal—pain. This way potential problems can be prevented or arrested early enough. This is especially important if the cause is congenital. The sooner you correct a weakness you were born with, the less damage or worsening of that condition will occur.

THE EVALUATION

Traditional procedures include: (1) examination of ortho-neurological tests designed to confirm the location of the source of pain as well as the degree of nerve involvement, (2) muscle testing to specifically identify areas of weakness, and (3) x-rays which act as a confirmation and as a visual aid (though discs, the major problem in many cases, do not appear on x-ray unless dye injections are included—a test performed by the orthopedist) and which later attest to results from manipulation. The true skill of the chiropractor is in his ability to palpate or touch the body and feel weaknesses, fixation of vertebrae, or other causes of trouble with his hands. All of these methods of evaluation are considered to diagnose the ailment.

The treatment has one goal in mind: to correct, strengthen, and rehabilitate the structure of the spine. Through hands-on manipulation, the chiropractor seeks to break up any muscle adhesions that have resulted from trauma, to stretch out contracted muscles supporting the back, and to reduce any vertebral displacement.

The chiropractor relies heavily on his techniques of manipulation, believing that treatment such as anti-inflammatory drugs or ultrasound are merely preliminaries to reduce pain. Chiropractic adjustments, as the manipulation is often called, are relatively safe, carrying minimal risks when compared to drugs or surgery. The schedule for a spinal adjustment varies with each individual and may continue for a period of months. Considering that your spine is suffering from ten to twenty or more years of abuse, such a treatment period may seem rather short compared to the results achieved.

In conclusion, the chiropractor is a practitioner who specializes in problems of the spine and the correct alignment of the body's structure in general, using hands-on manipulation as the preferred treatment.

THE OSTEOPATHIC PHYSICIAN (D.O.)

Most people—potential patients—have a great many misconceptions about the osteopathic physician, much of this being due to the medical doctor, or M.D.'s resistance to acknowledge the D.O. as a peer. The fact is, the training of both physicians is virtually identical. They take the same curriculum, the same test for licensing, and can treat patients, prescribe medication, and perform surgery as well. The greatest difference is that the osteopathic physician takes additional courses in the osteopathic field to learn the holistic approach that is synonymous with this branch of medicine, and to learn the hands-on manipulation and rehabilitation therapies so important in back care. In the words of one osteopathic physician, what is needed is some good public relations to get across the message of osteopathy, and not to assimilate it with other branches of medicine, which threatens to erase the uniqueness of the osteopathic philosophy.

The osteopathic branch of medicine grew from the frustration one medical doctor had with the way medicine took care of the disease, rather than the patient. Dr. Andrew Taylor Still founded the American School of Osteopathy in 1892, so it is a relatively new science. But the basic tenets of osteopathy couldn't be more at home than they are with today's emphasis on prevention. The osteopathic physician is trained to look at the "big picture"—the patient's whole environment—to better serve him. He believes that many external influences— work, family, friends, and coworkers, as well as eating habits, exercise, and the great influence of stress—are responsible for any given condition. In other words, treat the whole patient, not just the part that's sick. He also believes that by correcting negative influences—improving diet and exercise habits, relieving stress, and resting—the body can heal itself without the need for many drugs and other therapies. He also believes that a body with a well-balanced muscle and skeletal structure and with good neuro- and vascular alignment can indeed ward off disease.

The holistic approach of the osteopathic physician makes him interested in preserving good health. Eighty percent of all osteopaths are primary care family doctors, not specialists. Thirty-six percent practice in areas where the population is under 20,000. They can best be compared to the general practitioner who takes a vested interest in all aspects of the patient, knowing that total care is the best prevention.

THE EVALUATION

The first part of a visit to an osteopathic physician consists of a lengthy history-taking. The patient will be asked about childhood and adult illnesses, hospitalization, and medications; about any allergies or idiosyncracies; about his family, job, and personal interests. Many questions will be very personal, but that is the best way for the osteopath to get the vital personal history he needs for proper treatment.

The second part of the visit is an examination in the standing posture. The spinal curve will be checked for any abnormalities. The spine's range of motion will be tested and the osteopathic physician will look for any nerve problems or muscle atrophy. If the visit is due to a specific ailment, any pain that is felt will be relieved first, then any spasm.

The treatment for back pain includes stretching exercises, manipulation, the brief use of pain medication to interrupt the pain-spasm cycle, and instruction in proper comportment and correction of poor chairs, mattresses, or shoes that could be contributing to the problem. Rest, to allow muscles to repair themselves and to relieve the stress of everyday living, is an important part of treatment. So is nutrition (especially if being overweight is causing the back strain). Only in severe cases needing surgery would an orthopedist or neurosurgeon be called in.

In conclusion, osteopathic practitioners are licensed physicians and family doctors who believe in using a minimal amount of medication and believe in correcting external influences that may prevent the body's structural integrity from repairing itself.

THE ORTHOPEDIST (M.D.)

The orthopedic surgeon is a trained physician specializing in diseases of the musculoskeletal system. The orthopedist treats all problems associated with back pain, from muscle/ligament damage to severe cases of herniated discs, to other, life-threatening conditions such as tumors. Though he will often recommend conservative therapies (bed rest, the heating pad) in the cases of minor backache he sees, the orothopedic surgeon is often called in after other practitioners have determined that these nonradical treatments aren't sufficient and surgery is to be considered.

The orthopedist will often work in association with a physical therapist trained in hands-on rehabilitation techniques. A registered physical therapist is usually part of his "prescription" when he feels surgery can be avoided.

Most of the orthopedist's training centers on being able to diagnose the many anatomical causes of back pain, whether it be trauma to the back or a result of other ailments such as bone disease, disorders of the nervous system, or a disease of the chest, abdomen, or pelvic organs. As a medical doctor, he is a diagnostician learned in the areas of disease and cure.

THE EVALUATION

As a medical practitioner, the orthopedist relies on a battery of diagnostic tests to make a formal diagnosis. These can include blood tests, x-rays (including CT scans), myelograms (injection of dye into the spinal canal to help visualize neural structures), discograms (the less-frequent injection of dye into the actual disc), and a physical and internal exam to help locate the area of pain. A careful, detailed medical history of the patient is recorded as well as answers to specific questions designed to narrow down the possible causes of symptoms.

A conservative regimen will include noninvasive treatments such as bed rest, anti-inflammatory drugs, and heat. If necessary, the use of ultrasound or traction might be advocated. Once the painful condition subsides, a course of abdominal strengthening exercises and posture basics will be started. For some patients, corsets to hold the lumbar curve are ordered.

For more severe cases, new techniques might postpone or eliminate the need for surgery. Some patients are candidates for a treatment of enzyme injections designed to shrink herniated discs, thereby relieving the pain and pressure associated with the condition.

In conclusion, the orthopedic surgeon is a highly skilled medical doctor specializing in the conservative and operative treatments of bone ailments. He has at his disposal many conservative measures of treatment, including those by a physical therapist, which should be considered and attempted before surgery is prescribed. In general, conservative measures are exhausted prior to surgical intervention.

4

SMART MOVEMENT

Reaching for a book, lifting a package, lounging in bed on a Sunday morning—these activities of daily living as they are called, are second nature to us, often accomplished without the slightest thought. Unfortunately, the very movements we take for granted are the ones which, over a period of years, can do the most damage. The way you reach for that book, how you bend to lift that package, and how you position yourself in bed are all crucial to maintaining the physical integrity of your back and your entire body. Smart movement means just that: holding and moving your body the smart and healthful way.

The benefits of smart movement are numerous. Aesthetically, smart body movements are graceful, coordinated, and enhancing in that they show your body to its best advantage. Psychologically, a statuesque posture, a strong walk, and positive actions tell others how you feel about yourself and are excellent reinforcements of your self-image. From a physical performance point of view, smart movement is *efficient*, *effective* movement: when you walk properly, you also walk more quickly, getting to your destination sooner. From a physiological point of view, you move with less strain or wear-and-tear on your body.

Conversely, faulty body mechanics, or using the body incorrectly, can and often will cause painful conditions; and the longer you continue moving your body in a harmful way, the greater the likelihood of damage becomes. For example, bending over to tie a shoelace incorrectly puts pressure on your back. While doing this once won't cause immediate harm, repeated over a lifetime of shoe-wearing all the mini-assaults to the back add up. Their cumulative effect is aches-and-pains. Now multiply this by all the other incorrect movements you might be making and the result is serious trouble. The toll of faulty body mechanics is not limited to the back either. It can extend to vital joints and ligaments as well as the muscles. Smart movement therefore acts as a measure of prevention, the key to good health.

Of course there is no way to completely eliminate the stress the body lives with each day, but it can be reduced with your careful attention. To give you an idea of the various forces that act on the back during everyday activities, consider the following chart based on a study conducted by Dr. Alf Nachemson, a pioneer in this area. By monitoring the pressure on the third lumbar disc, the one most susceptible to damage, Dr. Nachemson measured the amount of force exerted on the back by a variety of movements. The eight common positions hold quite a few surprises.

THE NACHEMSON STUDY CHART

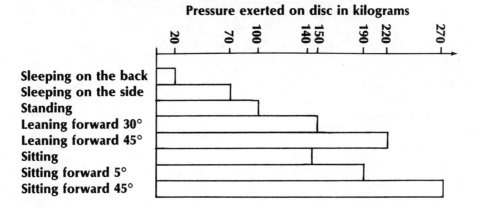

Pressure exerted on disc in kilograms

20   70   100   140 150   190 220   270

Sleeping on the back
Sleeping on the side
Standing
Leaning forward 30°
Leaning forward 45°
Sitting
Sitting forward 5°
Sitting forward 45°

As you can see from the chart, standing, for instance, is less stressful than sitting.

The conclusion? Pay strict attention to your posture and movements. Anytime you sit, sit correctly. Anytime you stand, stand correctly. To re-educate your motor senses, the following two sections offer the basics in comportment (how to *hold* the body) and in the activities of daily living (how to *move* the body).

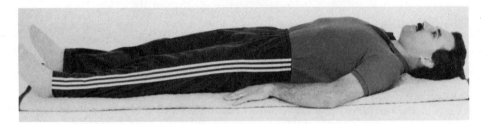

Sleeping on the back exerts 20 kilograms of pressure.

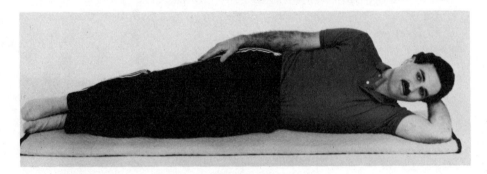

Sleeping on the side exerts 3.5 times the pressure of sleeping on the back.

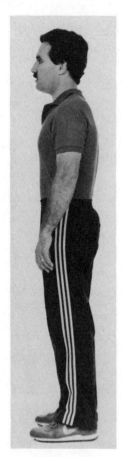

*Standing exerts 5 times the pressure
of sleeping on the back.*

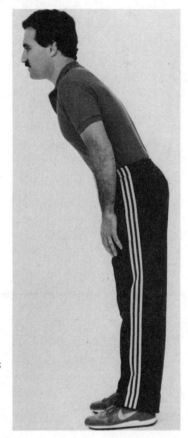

*Leaning forward at 30° exerts 7.5 times
the pressure of sleeping on the back.*

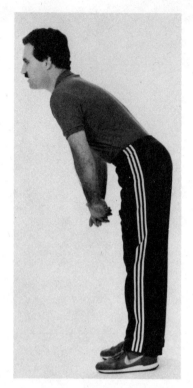

Leaning forward at 45° exerts 11 times the pressure of sleeping on the back.

Sitting exerts 7 times the pressure of sleeping on the back.

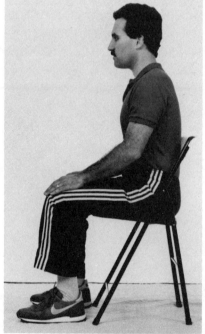

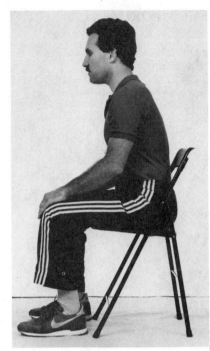

Sitting forward at 5° exerts 9.5 times the pressure of sleeping on the back.

Sitting forward at 45° exerts 13.5 times the pressure of sleeping on the back.

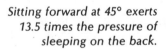

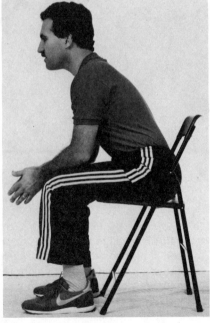

THE IMPORTANCE OF COMPORTMENT

STANDING TALL

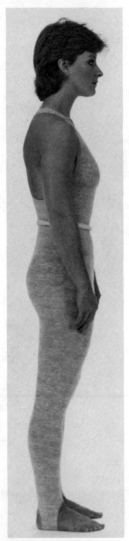

To stand correctly, first picture the curve of your spine which you want to maintain. Then align yourself accordingly: your head sits directly on your shoulders, eyes forward, chin parallel to the floor; your shoulders are straight and pressed back gently to remove any slump; your chest is up, but not forward, and in line with your ribs, waist, and hips; your arms are at ease along the sides of your body; and your legs are straight, feet slightly apart for balance.

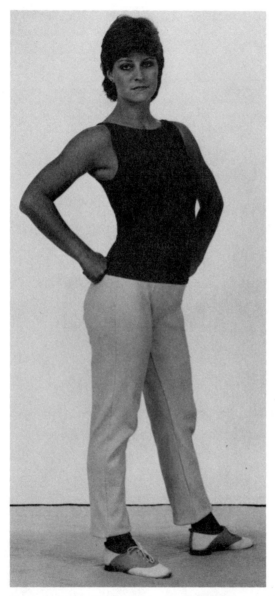

Poor posture is anything less than the previous description, but in particular, this haphazard stance not only looks ungraceful, but is also wrenching your back. Don't flatten or, at the other extreme, hyperextend your back or backside. Also resist crossing your ankles, a bad habit that throws off your balance and misaligns your body.

WALK THIS WAY

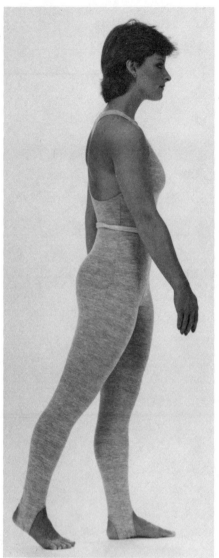

Maintain good standing posture with your chest held high and weight evenly distributed along both legs. Push off with the heel of the right foot to bring the left foot forward. Keep your head and torso up, maintaining the lumbar curve as you walk. Your legs, not the torso, do the work. Your arms may swing slightly.

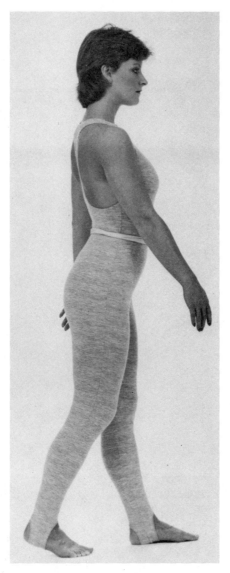

Do not lead with your shoulders, chest, or with hips thrust forward. Your arms should not propel you like oars.

SIT UP AND TAKE NOTICE PART ONE:
HOW TO SIT CORRECTLY

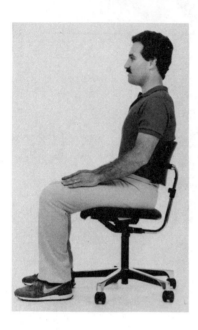

To sit properly, start with a chair that offers support for the back. The Giroflex chair, pictured here, is excellent, especially if you work long hours at a desk. Be sure to sit on the full seat.

Ideally, you should be able to adjust the seat to your body. Your knees should be higher or even with your hips.

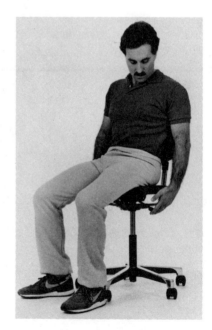

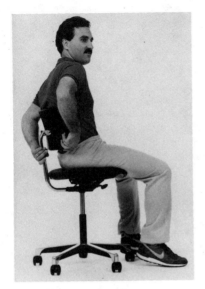

The back of the chair should also be adjustable to support your lumbar curve.

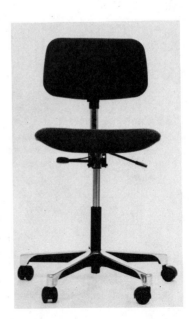

The Giroflex chair.

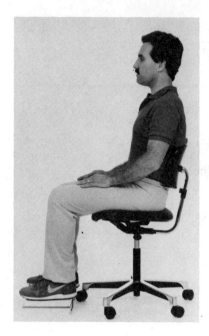

If your chair is too high for your feet to touch the ground with knees at the proper elevation, place a few books under your feet.

If you must cross your legs, do so at the ankles, not at the knees, which would pull the pelvis out of line and cause you to slip down in your chair.

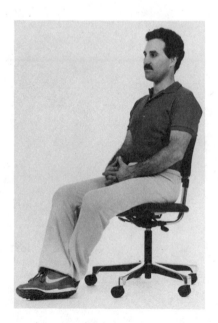

SIT UP AND TAKE NOTICE PART TWO: WHAT NOT TO DO

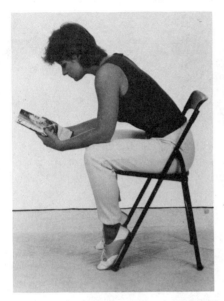

Don't lean forward with your elbows propped on your knees or a table. Though this position seems correct because the back looks straight, it is incorrect; you want to maintain the lumbar curve, not a flat back.

Don't slump backwards so that you are on the edge of a chair rather than properly positioned on the seat.

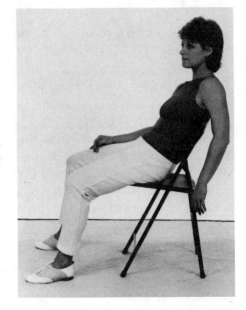

GETTING A GOOD NIGHT'S SLEEP

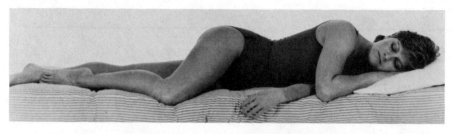

To sleep on your side, keep the bottom leg straight and bend the upper leg so that it lies away from your body on the mattress. This position takes the pressure off your back and preserves the lumbar curve. This is the optimal sleeping position.*

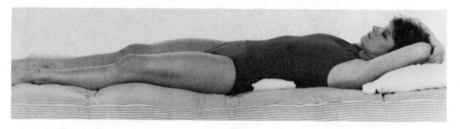

To sleep on your back, place a small, flat pillow under the small of your back to maintain the natural lumbar curve.

Special notes: A waterbed may be a qood option for some because the water supports the lumbar curve as it conforms to the shape of your body.

A too-soft mattress flattens the curve of the spine. Place a plywood bedboard between the mattress and the box spring for added firmness, especially if you sleep on your back.

Sleeping on the stomach is not a good idea for anyone because this position also discourages the natural lumbar curve.

---

*Do not confuse this modified side position with the one-leg-on-top-of-the-other side position which Nachemson showed put more strain on the back than lying flat.

BEDTIME STORY

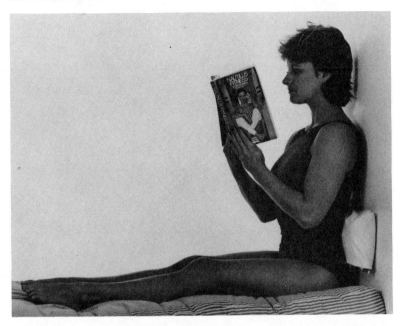

To preserve the lumbar curve when sitting up in bed, again use the small, flat pillow and place it between your headboard and the small of your back to simulate the support you'd get from a good chair.

GETTING UP ON THE RIGHT SIDE OF THE BED

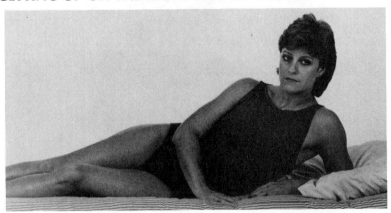

To get out of bed, turn your body towards the edge of the bed and prop yourself up on your side.

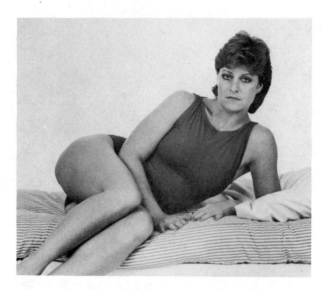

Swing your legs over the side of the bed.

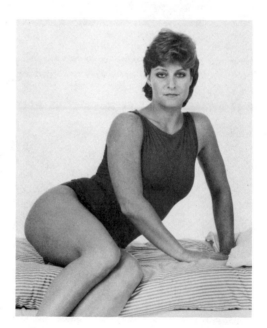

Use your hands to press yourself up to a sitting position.

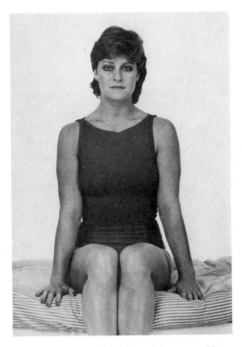

Then use your hands to lift yourself to your feet.

THE ACTIVITIES OF DAILY LIVING

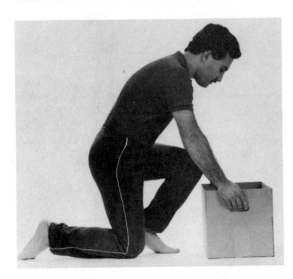

BENDING OVER

Do *lower yourself to one knee to pick up a heavy object, to empty the dishwasher, to check a roast in the oven, to arrange books in a low cabinet, or to retrieve one from a low shelf. (An alternate movement would be squatting.)*

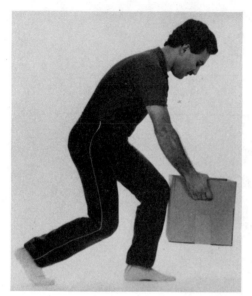

To lift from a kneeling position, press down on the foot of the raised knee to lift the other from the floor, the reverse of the movement for lowering yourself.

Press down on the heel of the lowered leg to straighten it fully.

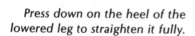

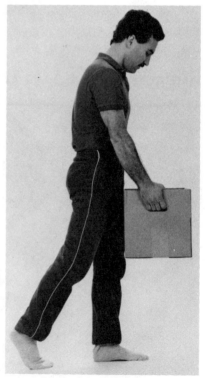

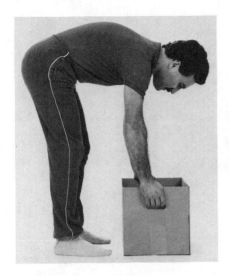

Don't *bend over from the waist as this not only disturbs the lumbar curve, but also strains the back muscles and stretches the ligaments that help hold the spine together.*

CARRYING

Below left: Do keep the object you are carrying close to your body. This forces you to use the muscles in your arms, legs, and abdomen. *Below, right:* Don't hold the object away from you. This incorrect movement forces your back muscles to do the work as it pulls your spine out of alignment to compensate for the weight.

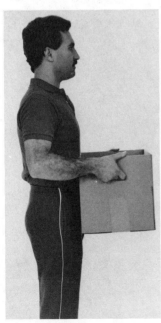
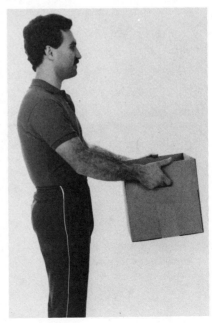

The Flying "A"

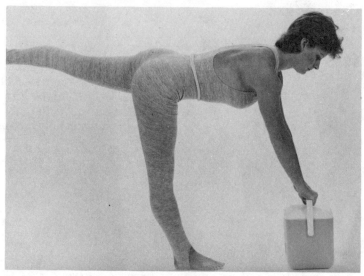

To lift a small or lightweight object, this movement is an alternative to kneeling. Press down on your right foot and use it as a hinge to raise your left leg behind you. Let your upper torso swing down to the floor, lowering your arms within easy reach of the object.

Working at a Table or Counter

Whether you are dicing vegetables in the kitchen, going over blueprints, or taking a phone message, the table or countertop surface should be high enough for your hands to reach from a standing position. Raise any free-standing tables to your level by placing equally thick books under the legs.

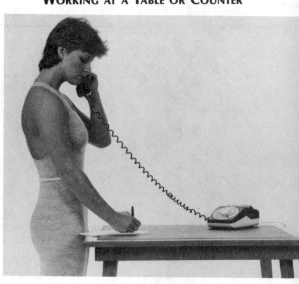

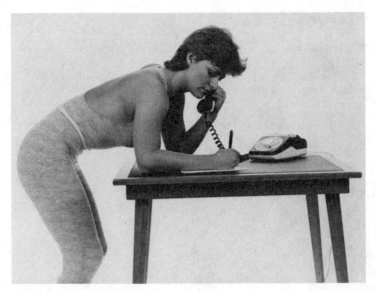

To compensate for a low, built-in counter, bend your knees to lower yourself.

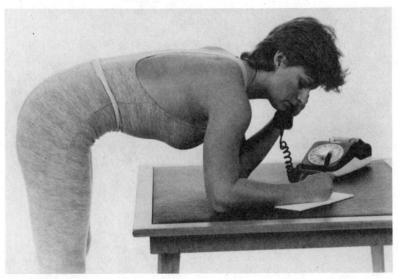

Do not lean over the table to accommodate yourself. Just look at what this does to the curve of your back and imagine the overstretching of the spinal ligaments.

Tying Shoelaces

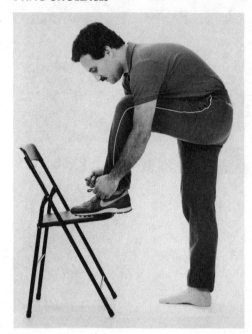

Do *raise your foot to within easy reach of your hands.*

Don't *bend over to bring your hands to your feet.*

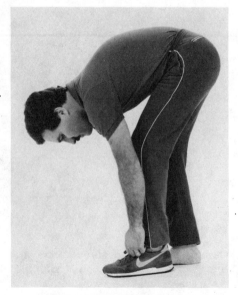

PACKING SUITCASES

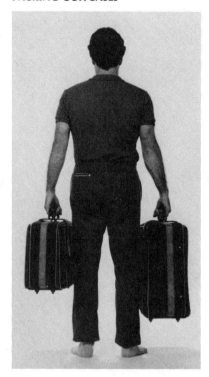

Do *use two small suitcases that are close to each other in size. Balance them by filling the smaller one, leaving the larger one slightly empty so that they weigh about the same when carried.*

Don't *overload one giant suitcase. Carrying a single object of great weight pulls your body out of line or causes you to overcompensate in the other direction.*

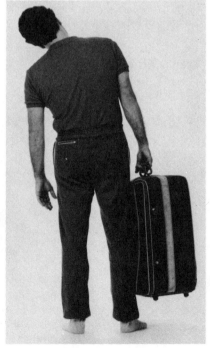

IRONING

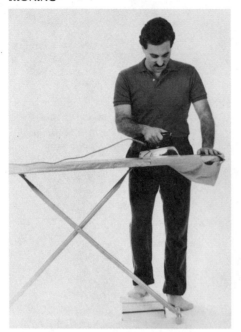

Do elevate one foot as you stand at the ironing board. This takes some of the pressure off your back when standing for prolonged periods of time. Note: whenever and wherever you find yourself standing, use your ingenuity to elevate one foot. At a bar, use the low railing designed for just that purpose; in the library stack, use one of the low stepstools.

SCRUBBING THE FLOOR

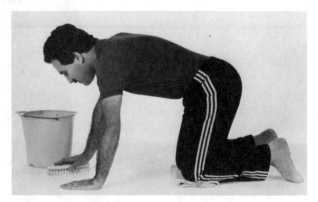

Do position yourself on all fours—the palms of your hands and your knees (with a towel under your knees to cushion them). Be sure that your head is in line with your spine. This will preserve the shape of your back to the extent that you can turn this photo on its side and note that my back looks like it is in the standing pose.

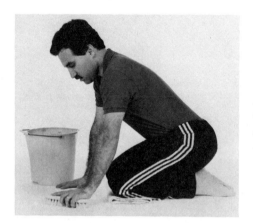

Don't *sit on your heels and stoop forward. This compresses your spinal discs and puts undue stress on the knees.*

FOR THE PREGNANT WOMAN

The weight gain from pregnancy places great stress on your spine. To compensate for this, especially in the second and third trimesters, pay extra attention to all the instructions for the activities of daily living and maintaining excellent comportment.

Resting, or taking short naps on your side periodically throughout the day will help alleviate tension in the back. By keeping your abdominal muscles strong, you help support the back naturally. Continue exercising them for as long as is comfortable, always with your doctor's consent. And when standing or sitting for long periods of time, be sure to change position often.

5

THE 20-MINUTES-A-DAY STRETCHING PLAN

Most people recognize the need for warm-ups before exercise, but did you know that you should warm up before you start your day? The best way to condition your back and body to make it healthier, more efficient, and better able to prevent stress and strain is with a 20 minute warm-up plan of light activity and stretches. Our program can loosen morning stiffness when you get out of bed and also relieve end-of-the-day fatigue when you get home from work or even before bed to ensure a restful sleep. The same stretches can also be repeated before any individual exercise program (especially the one we've designed in the next chapter).

Because the stretches are all leisurely and easy, it would be hard to overdo them. Two or even three times a day is fine, provided of course you have the time, but once a day is a must. Although it's best to perform the stretches in the morning, if your a.m. time is rushed as it is, by all means do them at night.

Follow these guidelines for maximum results.

1. Wear loose fitting clothing, or nothing at all. Tight garments can restrict your movement.

2. The first part of the warm-up plan calls for three to five minutes of an easy physical activity to actually warm the muscles. Contrary to popular misconception, stretching does not do this. (A sweet analogy: if you tried to stretch taffy candy when it's cold, it would break; to stretch it easily, you must first warm it.) Do 25 jumping jacks, or jog (but not run) in place, or walk the length of your living room ten times.

3. The second part calls for the program of stretches that follow. Stretching exercises the plastic element of your muscles which in turn determines your degree of flexibility. When you stretch, work slowly. Allow the full holding time to elapse before releasing a position, and then release it G-E-N-T-L-Y. Gradual movement is what works that plastic element and maintains flexibility.

4. If you are pressed for time, select eight to ten of the stretches and do them carefully. It's better to do a few of the stretches correctly (that means for the full holding time) than to race through all of them (an "exercise" in wasted time). Here is a good selection: stretches #3, #4, #7, #9, #11, #12, #13, and #14.

5. Take each stretch through a range of motion equal to or slightly beyond the range of motion required for the next part of your workout. Let's use running as an example. When you run, your legs work through a small range of motion, so there is no need to push each position to the maximum. However, if you were to follow your stretches with some swimming, with emphasis on the butterfly stroke which requires a great range of motion, you would take each stretch as far as you could comfortably.

The following program reaches all areas of the body including the hamstrings, the quadriceps, and the abdominals, as well as the muscles of the back. This is because the health of these other areas has a direct effect on the health of your back.

STRETCH #1: LATERAL FLEXION

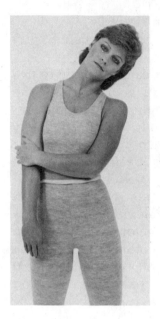

Hold your right elbow with your left hand and gently press it into your side as you stretch your head to the left. Hold this position for 20 seconds, then release. Repeat twice more to the left, then three times to the right.

STRETCH #2: LATERAL ROTATION

Place your left hand on your right shoulder as you rotate your head to the left. Hold this position for 20 seconds, then release. Repeat twice more, then three times on the other side.

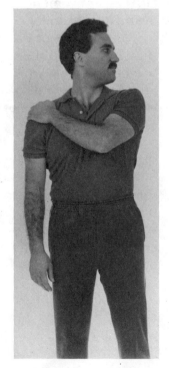

STRETCH #3: SIDE BEND

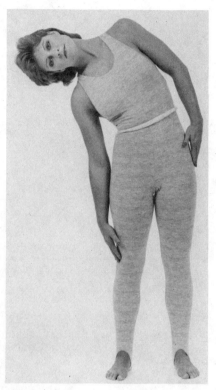

Stand with your arms at your sides. Without leaning forward or backward, lift up from your waist and lean your torso to the right. Hold this position for 20 seconds, then release. Repeat twice more, then three times to the left.

STRETCH #4: OVERHEAD REACH

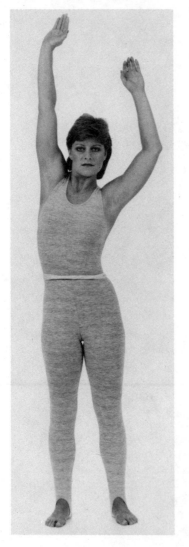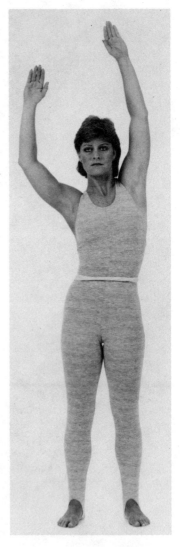

Stand straight with feet shoulder width apart. Raise both arms overhead, palms facing forward. Without leaning forward or backward, reach to the ceiling with your right hand, then with your left. Continue alternating arms in slow succession for 20 seconds. Relax for three seconds, then repeat for another 20. You should feel the stretch from waist to shoulder on either side.

STRETCH #5: REAR DELTOID (SHOULDER) STRETCH 1

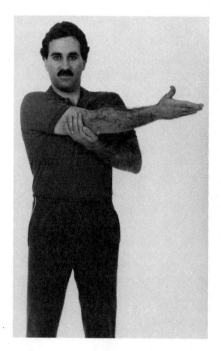

Bring your right arm across your chest and use your left hand to apply gentle pressure just above the right elbow. Hold this position for 20 seconds, then release. Repeat twice, then three times with the left arm across your chest.

STRETCH #6: DELTOID STRETCH 2

Stand facing a wall, your right arm outstretched and perpendicular to your body. With your shoulder touching the wall at all times, turn your body to the left. Hold this position for 20 seconds, then release. Shake out the arm and repeat twice, then three times with the left arm outstretched, body to the right.

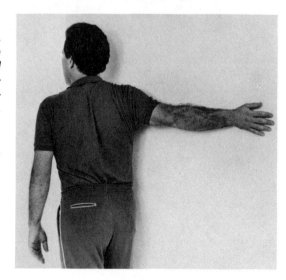

STRETCH #7: MEDITATION SIT

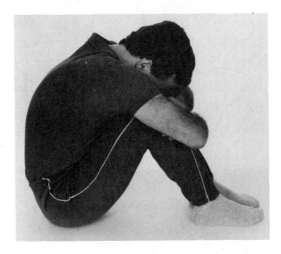

Sit on the floor with your knees drawn into your chest, arms hugging your legs. Lower your head to your knees to stretch your upper back. Hold this position for 20 seconds, then release. Repeat twice more.

STRETCH #8: SPINAL ROLL

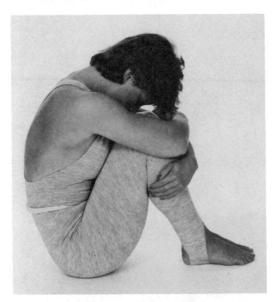

1. Start in the same position as stretch #7.

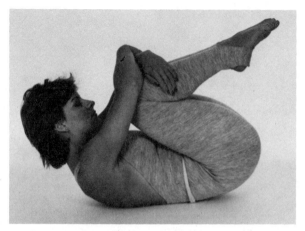

2. Slowly roll your spine back to the floor.

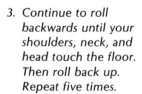

3. Continue to roll backwards until your shoulders, neck, and head touch the floor. Then roll back up. Repeat five times.

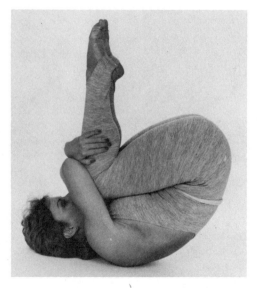

STRETCH #9: LOWER BACK STRETCH 1

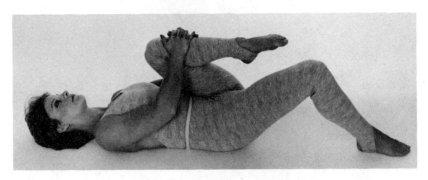

Lie flat on the floor and draw your left knee into your chest. Hold this position for 20 seconds, then release. Repeat twice more, then three times with the right leg.

STRETCH #10: LOWER BACK STRETCH 2

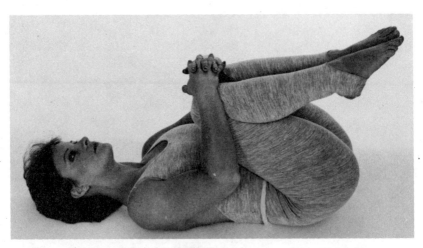

Lie flat on the floor and bring both knees to your chest. Hold this position for 20 seconds, then release. Repeat twice more.

STRETCH #11: SPINAL TWIST (PRONE)

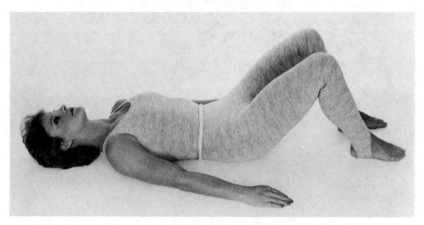

1. Lie on your back, knees bent, feet flat on the floor.

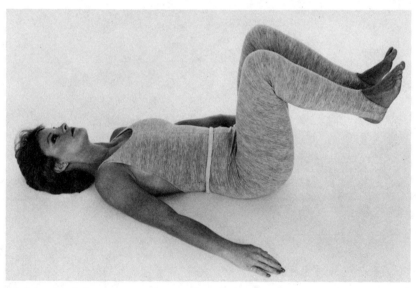

2. Bring both knees toward your chest.

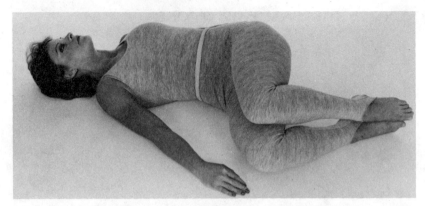

3. Keeping your shoulders and back pressed into the floor, twist at your waist to bring your knees straight to the floor on your right side. Hold this position for 20 seconds, then bring your knees back to the position in step 2. Repeat twice more to the right, then three times to the left.

STRETCH #12: SPINAL TWIST (SEATED)

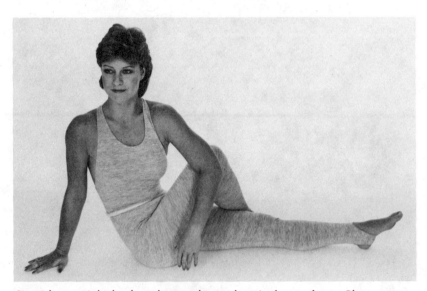

Sit with a straight back and extend your legs in front of you. Place your right ankle over your left leg so that the right foot is flat, with the ankle on the outside of the left knee. Turn your upper torso to the right and bring your left arm over the bent right knee. Keeping your shoulders pressed back, hold this position for 20 seconds, then release. Repeat twice more, then reverse all directions and repeat three times.

STRETCH #13: QUAD STRETCH

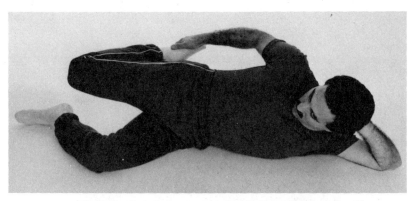

Lie on your side, legs slightly bent. Take hold of the top foot and press it back toward your buttocks, keeping the leg parallel to the floor. By applying pressure to the foot, work to press the foot as close to your buttocks as possible. When you feel the stretch in your thigh, hold the position for 20 seconds, then release the leg. Repeat twice, then roll onto your other side and repeat with the other leg.

STRETCH #14: HAMSTRING STRETCH

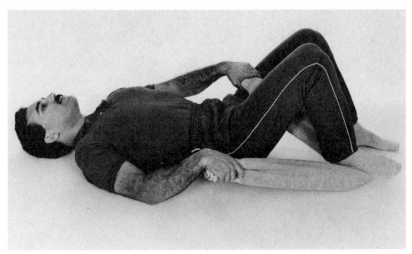

1. Lie on your back with your legs bent and feet flat on the floor. Wrap a towel under your right foot.

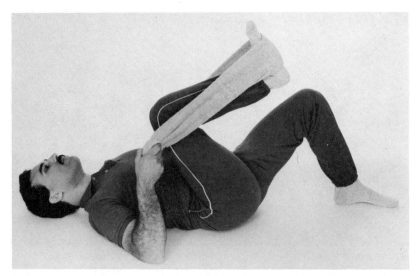

2. By exerting pressure on the towel, bring your right knee to your chest.

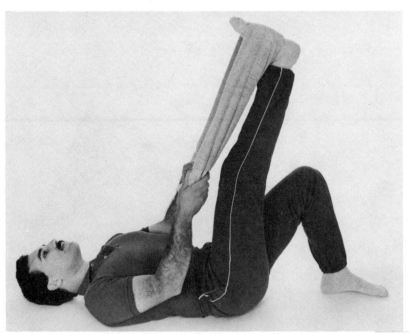

3. Slowly straighten the right leg toward the ceiling, only as far as you can comfortably go. Hold this position for 20 seconds, then release. Repeat twice more with the right leg, then three times with the left.

STRETCH #15: THE LOTUS

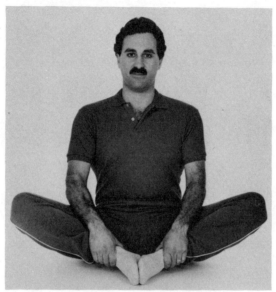

Sit with the soles of your feet together, knees pressed into the floor. Gently bring your heels as close to your body as is comfortable. Hold this position for 20 seconds, then release. Shake out your legs, then repeat twice more.

6

THE BETTER BACK
WORKOUT

The better back plan is an exercise workout to strengthen your body. It works not only the muscles of the back, but also the abdominals, the quadriceps, and the hamstrings. Strong abdominal muscles act as a firm girdle to support the back while you stand, walk, or lift. Strong thigh muscles enable your legs to carry much of the stress load that would otherwise fall on the back when you are climbing stairs, squatting (rather than bending over), or getting out of bed. Strengthening these muscles is the key to preventing a bad back or a painful reoccurrence of a back condition.

The better back workout should be incorporated into your fitness schedule at the rate of three times a week, practiced *after* you're fully stretched. The exercises are grouped by the various muscles which are worked. Within each grouping, the exercises are listed in graduating degree of difficulty. Depending on your physical condition you might be able to do all of them, or just the first exercise within each set. A beginner would do the basic curl-up, but not the variations; the single leg lift, called the "90-45," but not the double; the pelvic tilt, but not the bridge. That's fine. As weeks pass, you'll gain strength and be able to tackle the next level of each grouping.

We've incorporated isometrics (the holding part) into all our exercises. This is an underrated but extremely useful tool; it also prevents you from working too quickly.

Once you can accomplish all the repetitions in each exercise, you will need to provide a further challenge for yourself. A common misconception is that you should increase the number of reps. A better idea, one that is more time efficient (meaning you'll get better results in less time) is progressive resistance—literally adding weight. For example, when you reach the stage where you can do 20 leg lifts with ease, start doing them with ankle or lace weights. Begin with a light weight, about ½ to 1 lb. Add on in ½ to 1 lb. increments as you progress.

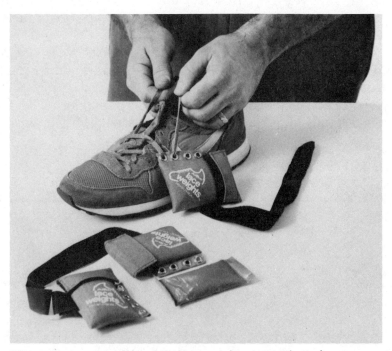

True to their name, these 1 lb. lace weights are easily tied onto your sneakers via their laces.

(*Note:* To those women fearful of adding bulky muscle, stop worrying. Highly developed muscles are achieved only with the help of testosterone, the male hormone. Since women have this in very short supply, it is nearly impossible to obtain muscleman proportions.)

To increase your resistance in exercises that don't readily lend themselves to the weights, or to add further resistance even to those that do, increase the length of the isometric phase of each exercise. For example: increase the holding time of the pelvic tilt from 5 to 10 seconds. A 3-second leg lift is held for 4, 5, or 6 seconds.

One caution: when doing each exercise, think of the natural lumbar curve of the spine. With each rep and with progressive action of the muscles, your body's natural tendency is to compensate with a reaction, often centered on the back. Therefore, if after any number of reps, especially with weights, you feel that you can't maintain the correct position of your back, stop. Exercise does strain the muscles, but should never cause pain or discomfort.

You should be able to see changes in yourself in as little as two weeks. Within a few months, the results should be great indeed. Be aware that some muscles will respond to exercise before others and that overall dimension changes will vary' from one individual to the next—that's genetic—but improvement is universal.

THE BETTER BACK WORKOUT

EXERCISE #1: GLUTEAL FLEXION

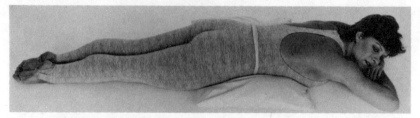

Lie on your stomach with a pillow placed under your abdomen. Pressing your pelvis into the pillow, squeeze your buttocks as tightly as you can. Hold for 5–10 seconds. Relax the muscles for 15 seconds. Repeat the entire exercise 3–5 times, building to 10.

EXERCISE #2: GLUTEAL LIFT 1

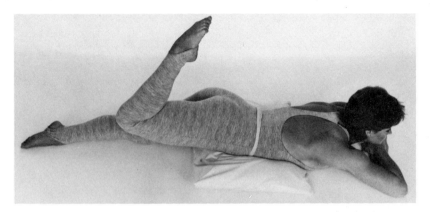

Starting in the same position, bend your right knee and lift the thigh off the floor. Hold for 5–10 seconds, then lower the leg. Repeat 5 times, building to 10, then repeat the entire exercise with the left leg.
Note: always keep the pelvis pressed into the pillows and the stationary leg straight.

EXERCISE #3: GLUTEAL LIFT 2

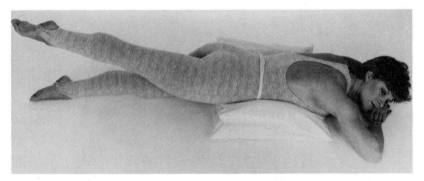

With two pillows under your abdomen, point your right foot and lift the leg slowly without putting an arch in your back. Hold this for 3–5 seconds, then lower the leg. Repeat 3 times, building to 10, then repeat the exercise using the left leg.

EXERCISE #4: GLUTEAL LIFT 3

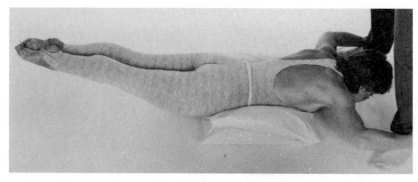

Holding a friend's ankles, or the legs of a solid table or chair, lift both legs simultaneously. Hold for 3–5 seconds. Repeat 3 times, building to 10.

EXERCISE #5: TORSO RAISES

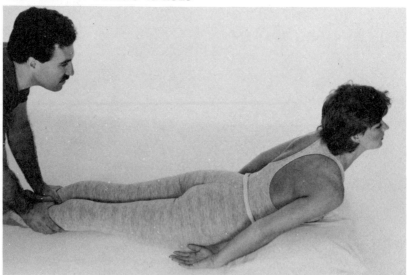

With a friend holding your ankles, or by locking your ankles around the legs of a solid table or chair, raise your head and upper torso without arching your back. Hold 3–5 seconds and lower. Repeat 3 times, building to 10.

EXERCISE #6: HAMSTRING PRESS

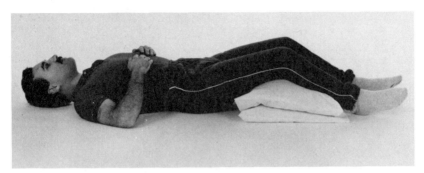

1. Lie on your back and place two pillows under your knees.

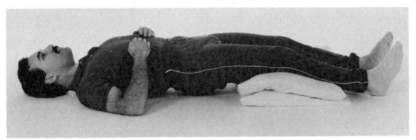

2. Press your knees into the pillows to straighten your legs. Your buttocks will raise slightly. Hold for 3–5 seconds, then relax. Repeat 3 times, building to 10.

EXERCISE #7: TUMMY TUCK

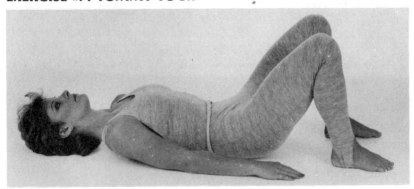

1. Lie on your back and bend your legs, feet flat on the floor, about six inches apart. Inhale.

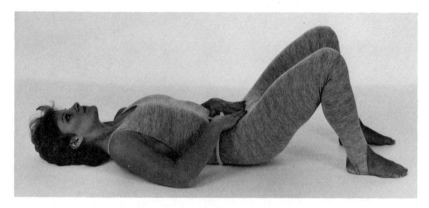

2. *Exhale and contract abdominal muscles. Think of trying to touch your stomach to your spine. Hold for 3–5 seconds and release, inhaling. Repeat 3 times, building to 20.*

EXERCISE #8: THE PELVIC TILT 1

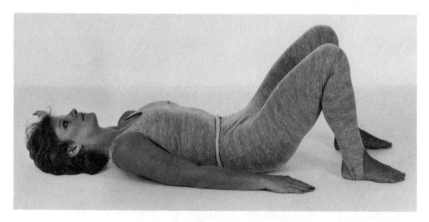

From the same starting position as exercise #7, press the small of your back into the floor and rotate your pelvis upward. Your buttocks contract to maintain the position and lift slightly off the floor. Hold for 3–5 seconds and release. Repeat 3 times, building to 20.

EXERCISE #9: PELVIC TILT 2

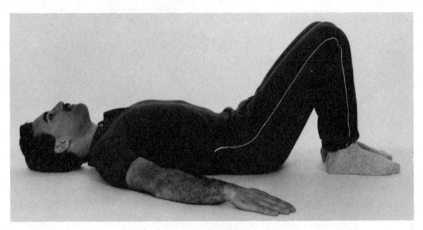

1. Start with your feet close to your buttocks.

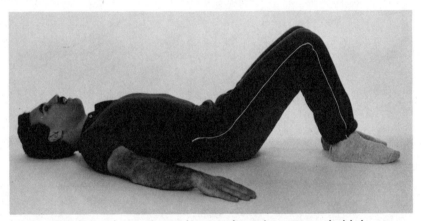

2. Contract buttock muscles and rotate the pelvis. As you hold the contraction, inch your feet forward.

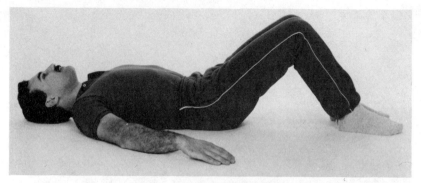

3. Continue moving your feet as far as you can go without losing the tilt contraction. Then slowly move your feet back to your buttocks to finish the exercise. Note: *you should spend 30 seconds moving your feet forward, 15 to move them back. This exercise is done only once.*

EXERCISE #10: THE BRIDGE

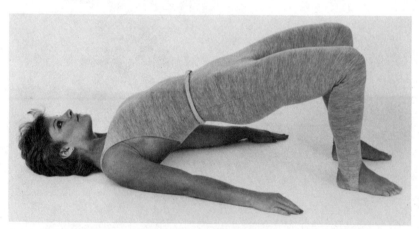

From the same starting position as in exercise #7, rotate your pelvis and contract the buttocks. Lift your bottom, then your lower back, and then your upper back off the floor until you are resting on your shoulders. You should feel the contraction the length of your thighs. Hold 5 seconds, then slowly lower in reverse order. Repeat 3 times, building to 20.

EXERCISE #11: CURL-UPS 1

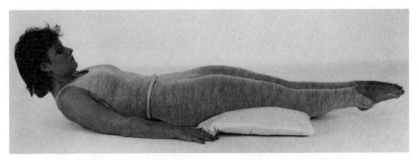

With a pillow under your knees—legs straight—lift your head and shoulders off the floor. Hold for 3–5 seconds, then lower. Repeat 3 times, building to 20.

EXERCISE #12: CURL-UPS 2

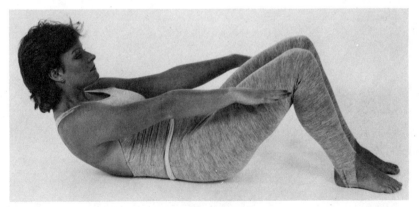

Remove the pillow and bend the legs, feet flat on the floor. Raise your head, shoulders, upper back, and arms. Hold 3–5 seconds, then lower. Repeat 3 times, building to 20.

EXERCISE #13: CURL-UPS 3

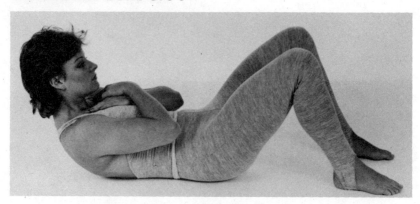

Repeat exercise #12 with arms folded across your chest.

EXERCISE #14: CURL-UPS 4

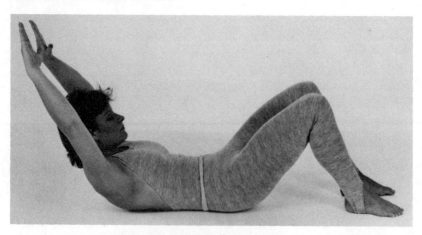

Repeat exercise #12 with arms extended overhead.

EXERCISE #15: CURL-UPS 5

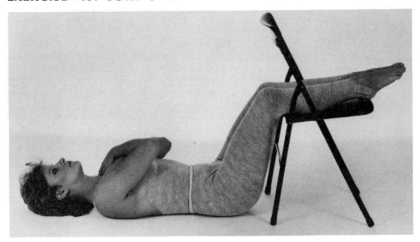

1. Raise your legs off the floor, with your calves resting on the seat of a sturdy chair.

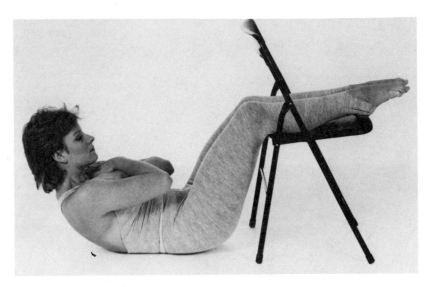

2. Curl up with your arms folded across your chest. Note: use same number of reps for exercises 13, 14, and 15.

EXERCISE #16: HEAD-TO-KNEE CURLS 1

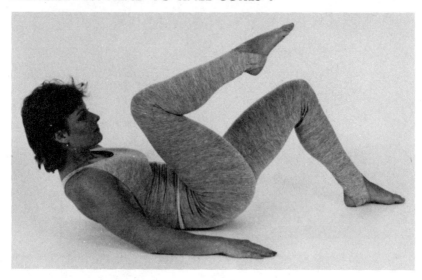

From the same starting position as exercise #7, simultaneously curl up head and shoulders and bring your right knee toward your forehead. Hold for 3–5 seconds, then relax to the floor. Repeat 3 times, building to 20, then repeat with the left knee.

EXERCISE #17: HEAD-TO-KNEE CURLS 2

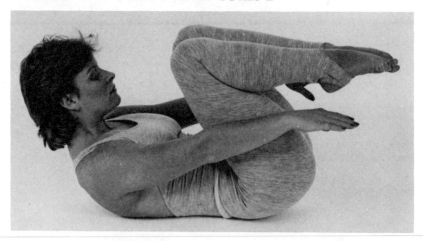

From the same starting position as exercise #7, simultaneously curl up head and shoulders and draw both knees toward your forehead. Hold for 3–5 seconds, then relax to the floor. Repeat 3 times, building to 20.

EXERCISE #18: LEG LIFTS

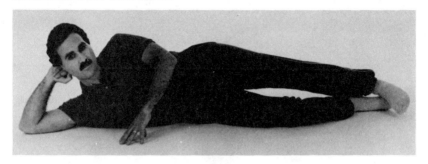

1. Lie on your right side, your right knee slightly bent for support.

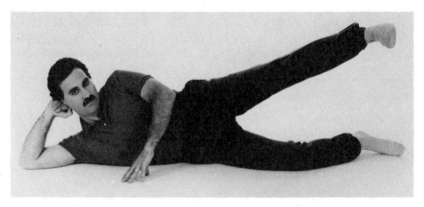

2. Keeping your left foot flexed, leg straight, raise the left leg as high as is comfortable. Hold 3–5 seconds, then lower. Repeat 8 times, building to 20. Repeat the entire exercise with your right leg.

EXERCISE #19: "90/45" LEG LIFTS 1

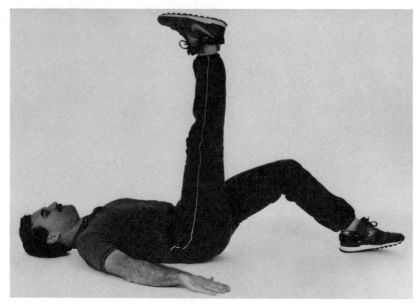

1. Lie flat on your back, arms at your sides. Keeping your left leg bent, foot flat on the floor, raise the right leg toward the ceiling to make a 90° angle with the floor.

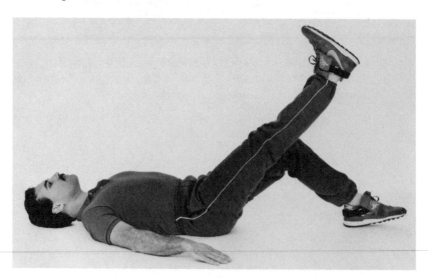

2. To a count of four, lower the leg halfway to the floor, making a 45° angle. Hold for 3–5 seconds, then bring the leg back up to the 90° mark. Repeat 8 times, building to 20, before lowering the leg. Then repeat the entire exercise using the left leg, right leg bent. Note: to increase difficulty, use weights as shown.

EXERCISE #20: "90/45" LEG LIFTS 2

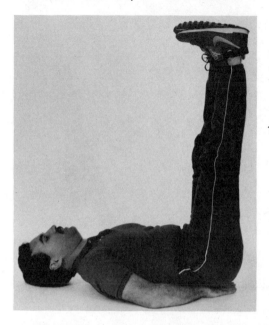

1. *Place your hands under your buttocks for support, then raise both legs to make a 90° angle with the floor.*

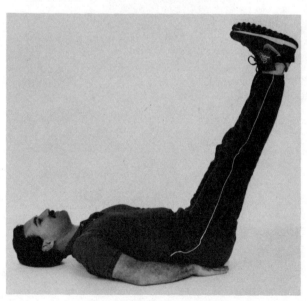

2. *To a count of four, lower both legs halfway to the floor, hold for 3–5 seconds, then bring them back to 90°. Repeat 8 times, building to 20.*

EXERCISE #21: DONKEY KICKS

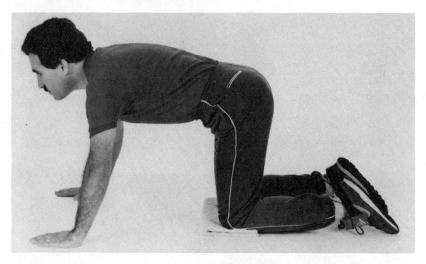

1. *Place yourself on all fours, palms flat on the floor, shoulder width apart. Cushion your knees with a towel, even if exercising on a soft surface.*

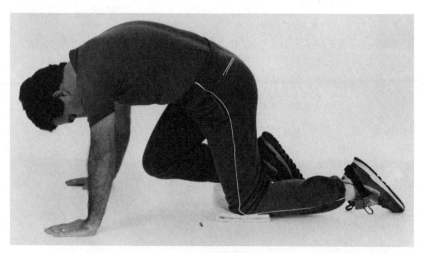

2. *Bend your head down and draw in your right knee toward your chin.*

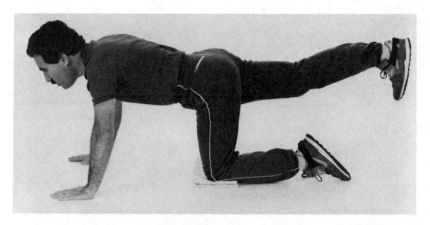

3. *Simultaneously lift your head and extend your right leg until it is level with your back, but not higher. Hold for 3–5 seconds while tightening gluteals. Then bring your knee back toward your forehead and repeat the kick 8 times without lowering the leg to the floor between kicks. Repeat the exercise using your left leg. Build to 20 times on each side.*

HOW TO COOL DOWN

After finishing these exercises (or any other activity), you must take the time to bring your body back to its usual state. End your workout by repeating those five minutes of light activity, then repeat the stretches. In other words, repeat your warm-up.

SPECIAL SPORTS INDICATIONS

Basic guidelines should be observed during other forms of activity to safeguard the back. When considering other exercises, think back to the Nachemson chart and evaluate the amount of stress to the back in relation to potential benefit to other parts of the body.

Use the indications that follow for specific activities.

CALISTHENICS

Avoid any movement that calls for you to touch your toes, especially with bouncing. This repeated assault on the spine causes compression of the discs and can damage the rear of the knees.

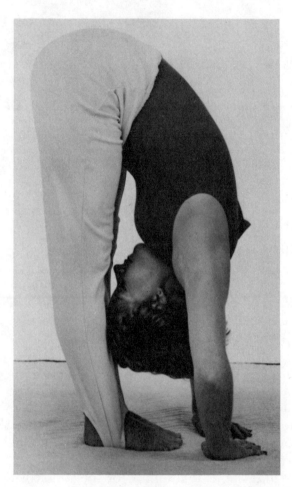

What not to do: Toe-Touches.

WEIGHTLIFTING

Avoid any deadlifts that cause you to bend over in the toe-touch position. This movement, compounded by the lifting of heavy weights, presses on the spine, dangerously compressing the discs.

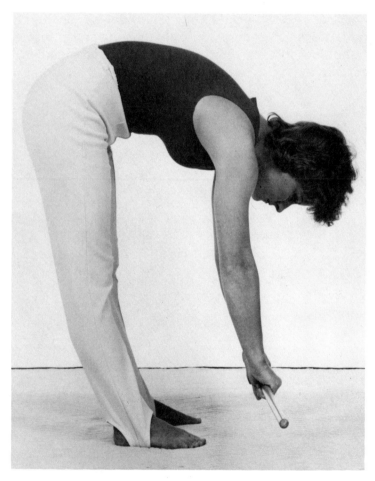

What not to do: Deadlifts.

YOGA

Slow, static stretching and the accompanying release of tension provided by yoga is great. But a few poses that threaten to take you past your limit of flexibility are dangerous. The plow, in which you throw your legs behind your head, can be especially damaging. In addition to compressing the spine, it cuts the flow of blood to the brain and can cause light-headedness or even fainting. Shoulder stands should be avoided as well. In general, do only those postures that keep your shoulder blades on the floor and that maintain the lumbar curve.

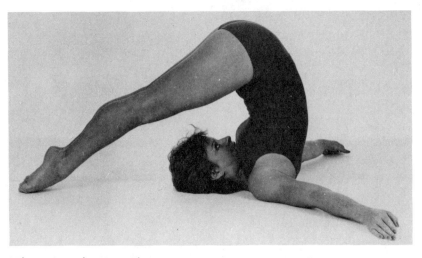

What not to do: Yoga Plow.

BALLET

This is a form of exercise that, taken in moderation, teaches you grace and control. However, too many participants try to be a Cynthia Gregory overnight, and too many teachers forget that their students don't have a ballerina's flexibility and years of training. The ballet barre positions ask too much of the novice; raising one's leg that high strains the all-important sciatic nerve. Stretching muscles is fine; stretching nerves is not. Keep your legs much closer to the ground or, better yet, try our safe hamstring stretch.

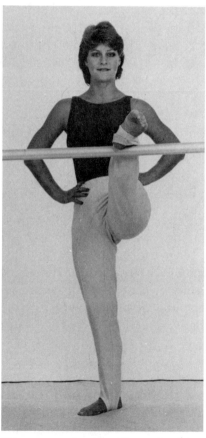

What not to do: Leg Lifts at the Barre.

CAUTIONS FOR AEROBIC ACTIVITY

RUNNING

This popular exercise greatly assaults the body. Consider that every time you land on one foot you do so at two to three times your body weight—200–400 lbs. of pressure riveting your body. To reduce the impact, the best running shoes on the market are a must. Think of them as an investment in your health, not just in footwear. The best running surface is the mini-trampoline, which absorbs all that pressure for you. Next in line, in order of preference, are: an indoor, cushioned track; a dirt road; or an asphalt surface, which has half the harshness of concrete.

(*Note:* to get all the benefits of running on the trampoline, be sure to keep a close check on your pulse and to vary the workout: alternate fast and slow jumps, ski twists, etc.)

JUMPING ROPE

Again, do it on a soft surface, wearing the best footwear. Start slowly and check your pulse often.

CYCLING

Be sure that your seat is high enough: legs should be almost straight when in the down position of the pedals. On the stationary bike, have the handlebars high enough to reach with a straight back. On an outdoor model, leaning over the frame is acceptable if most of your body weight is on your arms. Vary your spinal position every five or ten minutes to avoid undue fatigue.

SWIMMING

This is the best exercise from both efficiency and health points of view. The water buoys your body and reduces pressure to the spine. Just be sure to warmup fully.

CROSS-COUNTRY SKIING

Unlike the stressful impact of downhill skiing, this variation works the important muscle groups without compressing the spine. Indoor simulators are so successful that they are often part of the back patient's treatment.

ROLLER SKATING AND ICE SKATING

With good posture and balance, these are fine choices. For an aerobic effect, work to increase your endurance and check your pulse often.

AEROBIC DANCING

The problem with some organized classes run by dancers is the same as with ballet: instructors demonstrate movements that class members can't hope to do and certainly shouldn't attempt. If you need the structured atmosphere of a class, be careful if asked to assume positions that go beyond your normal range of motion.

INDEX